CW00381878

HUMAN BIOMECHANICS OPTIMIZATION FOR AGING BACKWARDS

SCIENCE BEHIND OVERCOMING POOR POSTURE AND GRAVITY (POSTURE CORRECTION BOOK)

BY RANGNATH GOUDA(POSTURE GURU)

This book was published thanks to free support and training from:

EbookPublishingSchool.com

TABLE OF CONTENTS.

Chapter 12. Rounded shoulders + Uneven shoulders + uneven shoulder height.

Chapter 13. Understanding and correcting uneven pecs, uneven traps, uneven lats and shoulders.

Chapter 14. Understanding and correcting Lateral pelvic tilt and twisted core.

Chapter 15. Training the nervous system with Stretching and strengthening exercises

Chapter 16. Mastering the Plank exercise.

Chapter 17. Conclusion

INTRODUCTION

My Name is Rangnath Gowda and also called as posture guru. I had a history of poor posture and muscle imbalance and in this book I am sharing all my knowledge of what I did to overcome my posture issues. I tried consulting a Physiotherapist, personal trainers and even at some point orthopedic doctors, but it was of no use because nobody knows how to fix it. I have spent almost 5 years researching how to fix posture or muscle imbalance issues. After doing the research I came to know the science behind human biomechanics and the fastest and easiest way of fixing postural problems. In this book you can read the science behind human biomechanics and how you can utilize this science to optimize your body for better posture by identifying and eliminating muscle imbalance.

 I have a blog https://posture-guru.com you can check out my post which may be useful for you from coming out of your postural issues. I also provide online consultation. You can mail me your request at postureguru7@gmail.com . For any queries or help please feel free to mail me or comment on my blog i will be happy to answer.

CHAPTER 1.INTRODUCTION-NEED FOR

OPTIMIZING THE HUMAN BODY

When a baby is born it has no control on its muscles, no past memory in its brain and no programming in its nervous System. Everything is in learning and adapting mode. In the age between 1 to 5 years it will start gaining the control over the muscles and then the baby can walk, run and can play with having complete balance and control over his body but at this age we don't develop postural problems except if there is some vitamin deficiency or structural problem which can bend the spine and can cause scoliosis. Here we are not going to discuss such postural distortions but, caused due to Stress and the increasing weight plus gravity on our body.

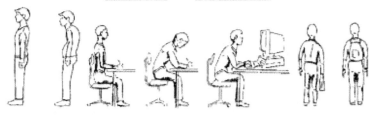

Figure 1 Common causes of poor posture

As we grow we start to develop stress on our body in different ways. Our weight starts increasing and the effect of gravity also starts increasing. Starting from the weight of the school bag on your back to slouching while sitting, these are the small causes of poor posture or bad posture but have a major impact in the long term. With the advancement of technology, millions of people are suffering from poor posture each year. Unfortunately, bad posture may lead to many health complications including spinal dysfunction, joint degeneration, respiratory problems and high blood pressure, among other things which leads to faster aging of the human body. By understanding the causes of bad posture and working to correct them, many of these posture-related conditions can be fixed But Question is " Is it ever possible to avoid or correct this postural distortions " and the answer is yes. which i call as to optimize our body to have better posture and as you read this book you will come to know how. Before knowing how?, we need to understand the causes of bad posture and its consequences

CHAPTER 2.CAUSES AND ITS CONSEQUENCES OF BAD POSTURE

a) **Carrying heavy weight on one side** - Carrying a heavy bag or purse on one side of the body leads to an imbalance in posture. It also presses muscles and nerves in the neck which run down to the shoulder and are severely strained due to constant load. If proper care is not taken in time, it can lead to frozen shoulders and arthritis. "Cumbersome bags may leave you with back, neck, and shoulder pain, even headaches, and can aggravate the arthritis conditions.

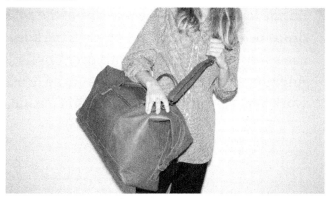

b) **Desk Job** - The wrong chair, improper desk setup (including poor monitor height) and lack of breaks can all contribute to keeping our spines straight in the workplace. On average, people are sitting at their desk jobs with their neck and head forward and shoulders hunched for more than nine hours a day.

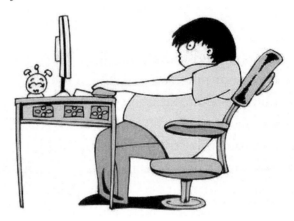

c) **Leaning or Standing on one leg** - When you lean on one leg while standing one side of the pelvis drops below the other. This stresses the knee and can contribute to osteoarthritis over time. Additionally, the lumbar spine has to go to extra work to ensure that the torso stays in position.

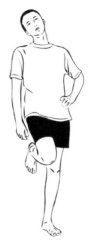

d) **Dominant one side of Body-** Everyone use there one side of their body more compared to Other side if it goes on increasing this creates imbalance in the body that causes unequal weight distribution on the spine and you may have to face asymmetrical postural problems leading to different body joint pains

e) **Isolated workouts/Exercises-** If we train one muscle at a time it creates unequal tension in the chain of muscles and creates imbalances in the muscles which leads to joint injuries or muscle strains. I know this point is difficult to understand but it will be clear once you read this book completely.

Chapter 3.Human Biomechanics

OPTIMIZATION

"Human Biomechanics Optimization is a process of aligning the body so that our centre of Gravity is Improved and we have less effect of gravity on our body which leads to Equal distribution of weight throughout our Body means achieving balanced tension in the muscle skeleton system".

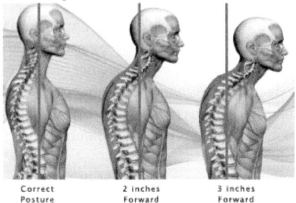

Did you know...?

| Correct Posture | 2 inches Forward | 3 inches Forward |

'For every inch (2.54cms) of Forward Head Posture, it can increase the weight of the head by an additional 10 pounds (4.54kgs)'

From the above picture you can see that even if our head is misaligned or is forward it can increase the weight on the spine which increases the curve of the spine. If you have an excess curve in the spine it will cause difficulty while breathing and if you don't inhale oxygen in the right proportion it will cause lower energy levels making you feel lazy or less energetic.

So how can we optimize our body ?

Do you know what tensegrity is?

Let's first understand the tensegrity before we understand How we can optimize our body.

Chapter 4. Understanding the tensegrity model and applying tensegrity principle to human body

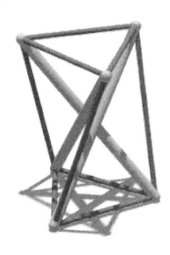

Tensegrity, tensional integrity or floating compression is a structural principle based on the use of isolated components in compression inside a net of continuous tension, in such a way that the compressed members do not touch each other and the prestressed tensioned members delineate the system spatially.

If you have not understood tensegrity i will explain it in an easy way with the help of the diagram below but i still recommend you go on and do research on the internet to get it more clear .

Below is the diagram of a tensegrity structure which consists of rigid rods and elastic bands that are under tension so that the entire system is stabilized.

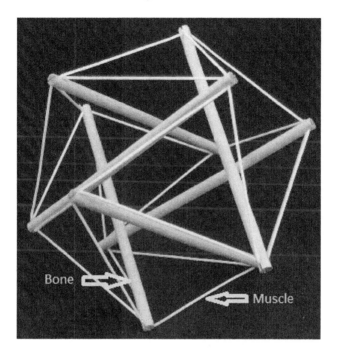

If we relate this structure to a human body the rods will be our bones and the elastic bands will be our muscles. if any of the elastic bands gets elongated the entire system undergoes a change. So if I want to relate tensegrity to the human body, if there is muscle imbalance (Lengthening or shortening of muscle) in one muscle also this will affect the entire body.

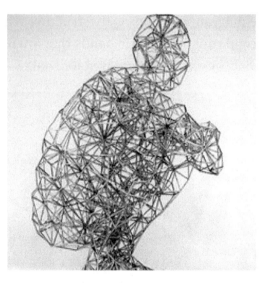

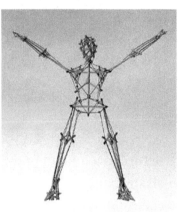

Figure 2Tensegrity model of human body

(<u>Search on internet for Better understanding of tensegrity model of human body</u>)

CHAPTER 5. SCIENCE BEHIND THE WORKING OF HUMAN BODY

Human body works in integration and most of the movement made by humans is walking and running so from this movement we can understand how the human body works. When we take our first foot while walking there are chain or muscle slings working together to create the movement efficiently. Our body never works in isolation but we train our muscles in isolation which is the reason for muscle imbalances which leads to poor posture and Injuries. Let's understand the different myofascial slings which promote the different movements. Before that lets understand reciprocal inhibition.

Principal of reciprocal inhibition

"When one muscle contracts the antagonist or the opposing muscle relaxes" Example when you flex the bicep muscle the antagonist muscle triceps relax or lengthens is called reciprocal inhibition.

Once you understand the principle of reciprocal inhibition, let's understand with an example .

Suppose you have a bad habit of leaning on one leg, let's see what happens to the entire body because of leaning on one leg.

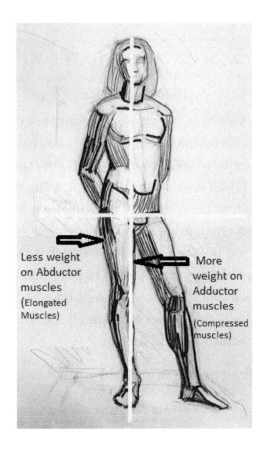

Less weight on Abductor muscles (Elongated Muscles)

More weight on Adductor muscles (Compressed muscles)

When you lean on one leg your center of gravity is shifted and most of your body weight is supported by one leg. from the above figure you can see that the most of the upper body weight is supported by the right leg and there is more weight on the adductor muscles which are under compression and in shortened state and the abduction muscles are in lengthened state on the right side this will create tilting of your upper body which will create muscle imbalances in the upper body. In order to understand how muscle imbalance occurs in the upper body we must first understand the Myofascial sling systems in the human body.

CHAPTER 6. GROUP OF MUSCLE CHAINS IN HUMAN BODY

What is Myofascial sling?

The sling is a group of contralateral (opposite) muscle groups that work in a diagonal fashion and that lie on the anterior (front) and posterior (back) portion of the trunk. The sling can be broken down into the posterior and anterior oblique slings. The primary function of the sling is to stabilize the pelvis and spine during movement, which enhances performance in all sports from track & field, football, baseball, golf and volleyball.

There are 4 key muscular slings:

○ The anterior oblique sling

○ The posterior oblique sling

○ The lateral sling

○ The longitudinal sling

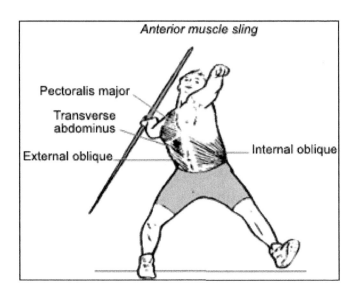

Anterior Oblique Sling

Whenever you make any kind of throwing or pushing movement with one hand it involves Anterior oblique sling muscles as in the picture shown. <u>So if I want to relate this to muscle imbalance, if you have a right side chest more stronger you will also have strong right side external oblique, left side internal oblique and left side adductor muscles.</u>

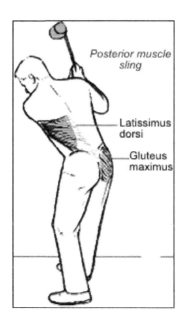

Figure 4 Posterior oblique sling

Posterior oblique sling helps us in pulling movements . or taking a long stance back while hitting a golf ball. The movement involves Latissimus dorsi and glute muscles.

So if i want to relate with a person having strong lats muscle on one side he will definitely have strong glute muscles on the opposite side.

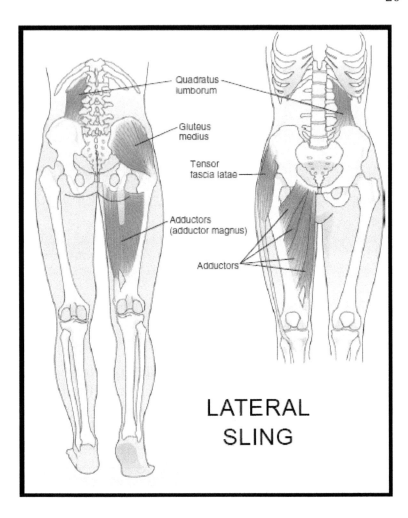

Figure 5Lateral sling

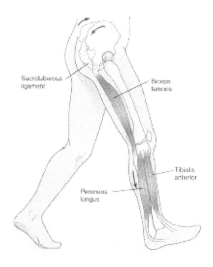

Figure 6 Longitudinal sling

Once we understand how our body movement works now let's see the different types of bad posture and know the weak and dominant muscles involved.

CHAPTER 7. IDENTIFYING OR FINDING MUSCLE IMBALANCES

Almost everyone on the planet has muscle imbalances and nobody has a completely balanced body. We use one side of our body mostly the right side and we never use both sides of our body equally, and we cannot identify the minute muscle imbalances in our body, but this minute muscle imbalances if not identified in the beginning will become big in future causing your entire body to imbalance and will lead to body joint pain and to overcome the pains you have to take tablets, medicinal drugs which will have side effects on human body.

So let's see how we can identify muscle imbalance.

Check list (Self assessment)

1) **Sweating More on one side:** Have you ever noticed your body keenly when you have done exercises and you start to sweat and you find that your right side of your arm is more watery (Sweaty) compared to left. This is a sign of muscle imbalances and your nervous system is focusing more on the stronger side.

2) **Cracking of your Jaws (Temporomandibular disorder):** Does your jaws make cracking sounds especially when you wake up in the morning or while sleeping. If your jaws get locked and you are

unable to open your mouth completely then this is the sign of muscle imbalance. Imbalanced body causes the spine to rotate and your jaws will be out of line causing instability.

3) **Feeling more weight on one leg:** Have you ever noticed you had a long run and you are tired and suddenly you start to feel more weight on one side of your body. This is a sign of muscle imbalance.

4) **Externally rotated hip or leg:** Does one of your legs externally rotate more compared to the other in supine position. This is an early sign of muscle imbalance and if not addressed earlier soon your entire body will be imbalanced.

5) **Uneven Expansion of ribs while breathing:** Have you ever noticed keenly by closing your eyes, holding your navel in and taking a deep breath and finding that one of the sides of your body is expanding more compared to other. Muscle imbalance causes your body to expand unevenly and it's the quickest and easiest way to identify weak muscles in your core because the weaker side expands more than the stronger side.

If you have done these above checks and find yourself matching with above symptoms then most probably you are in a stage where you will have body joint pains in future and if not corrected and you are involved in high intensity weight lifting activities you may have a chance of getting injured.

Chapter 8. Importance of the body form while doing exercises

You must have noticed that whenever you go to any gym and you hear from the trainers that you should always maintain a proper form while doing exercises or else you may get injured. I agree that you may get injured but most important is that it will create muscle imbalances in your body and if you do not maintain your spine straight then your center of gravity will be shifted and your muscles will be pulled in the direction of the shifted center of gravity.

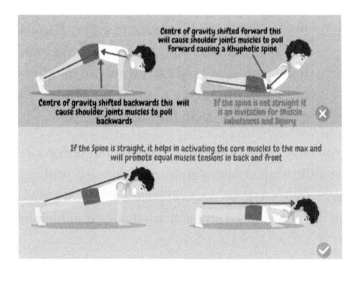

Another effect of bad form is that if your spine is not straight while doing any exercise then it becomes difficult for your body to stabilize your spine and you will face difficulty in activating the core muscle i.e transverse abdominis which helps in stabilizing the spine keeping it neutral.

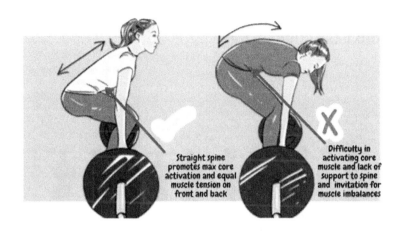

Straight spine promotes max core activation and equal muscle tension on front and back

Difficulty in activating core muscle and lack of support to spine and invitation for muscle imbalances

Chapter 9. Common bad postures and quick fixes

As per Google Muscular imbalance occurs when one muscle is stronger than its opposing muscle. Its half correct muscular imbalance occurs when a group of muscles are stronger than its group of opposing muscles as we know that human body works in integration and not in isolation

Once we know the type of posture we have or once we know the weak and strong muscles then we can Take first step to correct the posture by stretching the strong muscles and strengthening the weak muscles

DIFFERENT TYPES OF BAD POSTURE ITS ASSESSMENT AND EASY CORRECTION

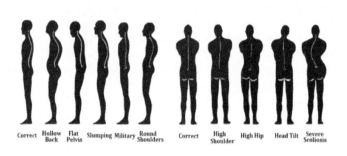

Correct Hollow Flat Slumping Military Round   Correct High High Hip Head Tilt Severe
         Back   Pelvis   Shoulders   Shoulder   Scoliosis

1) Hollow back Posture

From the picture you can clearly see that you have weak lower abdominal muscles and strong upper abdominal muscles. If you look at the antagonist muscles, hyperextended lumbar spine and slouched upper back which leads to weak thoracic spine muscles. Correction is that you need to stretch the strong muscles and strengthen the weak muscles as we know now the strong and weak muscles.

2) Flat pelvis posture and slumping posture

Flat pelvis posture is also called a posterior pelvic tilt. It is caused due to overdeveloped glutes muscles and weak hip flexors in the lower body and strong abdominal muscles, strong chest muscles and weak back muscles. It is the result of sitting in a slouched posture. Men are more prone to flat pelvis posture. Strengthening back muscles and hip flexor muscles will help to reverse this type posture condition.

3) Military posture

According to me, military posture is not that bad a posture condition that you need to worry about. It is caused due to sitting in an erect state and having strong back muscles and weak abdominal and chest muscles. It's completely okay to have military posture until you don't have any kind of pain . Strengthening the core muscle will help in fixing the issue.

4) Rounded shoulders posture.

It is caused due to sitting in a slouched state in front of computers or training more chest muscles. Stretching

the chest and anterior shoulder muscles will fix this
condition easily.

Back extension exercise for rounded shoulders

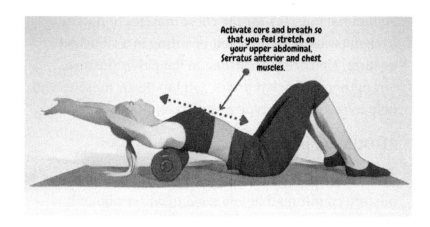

**Exercise to stretch front muscles and strengthen back
muscles**

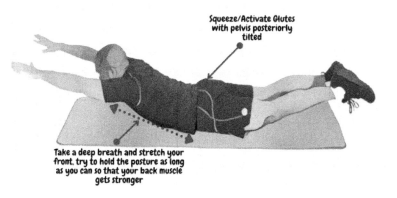

Squeeze/Activate Glutes with pelvis posteriorly tilted

Take a deep breath and stretch your front, try to hold the posture as long as you can so that your back muscle gets stronger

5) Asymmetrical shift or asymmetrical posture

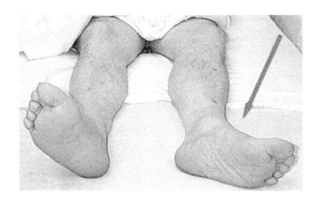

Figure 7 externally rotated leg

If you have an Asymmetrical posture there is a high chance of one of your legs externally rotated and also the vice versa, If you have one sided externally rotated leg then chances are you are going to develop asymmetrical posture in future or may have it. A person with Asymmetrical posture will have muscle imbalance in his entire body. In the picture (Fig.8) you can see that one of the shoulders is high compared to the other shoulder and one side hip is high. In this case you have one side anterior oblique muscles stronger and strong posterior oblique muscles on the other side. so to fix it we need to stretch the both contralateral oblique chain of muscles.

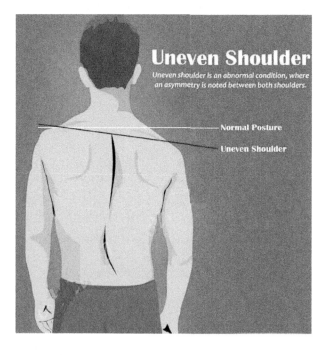

Figure 8 Uneven shoulder heights

Shoulder on the lower side is pulled forward and lowered by the strong external obliques and the lats on the same side is weak and

unable to pull back the shoulders. Also the trapezius muscles are also weak on the same side.

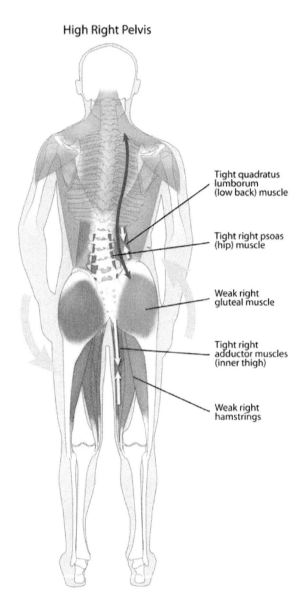

Figure 9 Asymmetrical posture

Signs of asymmetrical posture

1)   Uneven chest muscles

2)   Uneven shoulder height and uneven traps.

3)   Leg length discrepancy

4)   S-Curve in the spine

5)   Uneven hips

6)   Uneven lats

7)   Feeling more weight on one side of the body

8)   Externally rotated leg

9)   Lower back pain

10)   Shoulder joint pain

11)   Temporomandibular disorder (TMD or TMJ)

CHAPTER 10. IMPORTANCE OF CORE IN FIXING POSTURE ISSUES

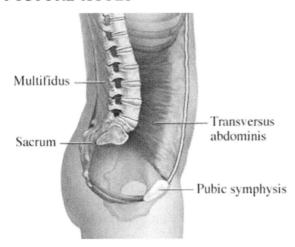

Multifidus

Sacrum

Transversus abdominis

Pubic symphysis

Figure 10 Core

Core is in between the thoracic rib cage and lumbo pelvic hip complex and imbalances In the hip muscle will travel up throughout the upper body so imbalance in hip will cause imbalance in the Thoracic muscles. Core holds these two portions of the body so if the core is stronger it will support the Spine and protect from muscular imbalances and poor posture. Stronger the core muscles better will be your posture

CHAPTER 11. FUNCTIONAL LEG LENGTH

DISCREPANCY AND ITS CORRECTION

Have you ever felt or noticed your leg shorter? If it is not a limb length discrepancy where the bone itself is short compared to other then you fall under the functional leg length discrepancy and the most important point you need to know is that your leg is not shorter actually but it appears as shorter.

Self assessment checks

If one of your hips or leg is externally rotating more compared to other then yes it's a sign that your externally rotated leg will appear shorter.

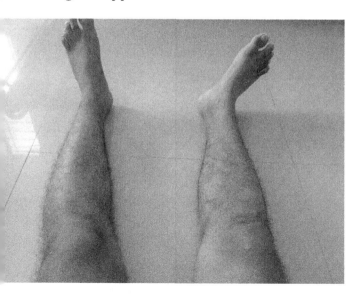

Knee height check

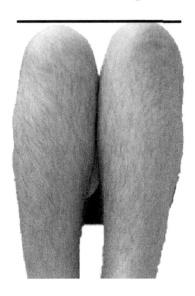

When you check your knee height in a sleeping position and after bringing your knees closer, you will find that the externally rotated leg is smaller.

Correction for functional leg length discrepancy

If your doctor says to use a shoe lift for correcting your discrepancy I would say not needed unless it is a real limb length discrepancy where there is no other option to use shoe lift. But in case of functional leg length discrepancy you need to stretch your abductor muscles and hip extension muscles of your externally rotated hip that includes Glutes and hamstring and you need to stretch the adductors and hip flexors of the other leg. After doing the stretching exercises you need to do a plank exercise so that your body adapts the changes made. Once you notice your legs are balanced you can stop the exercises.

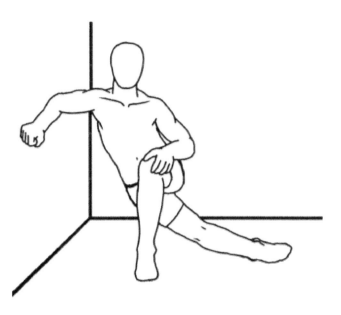

Abductor muscles stretch

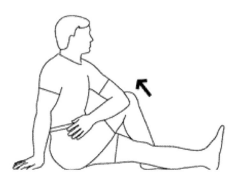

Glutes Stretch

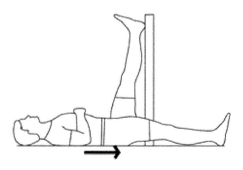

Hamstring wall stretch

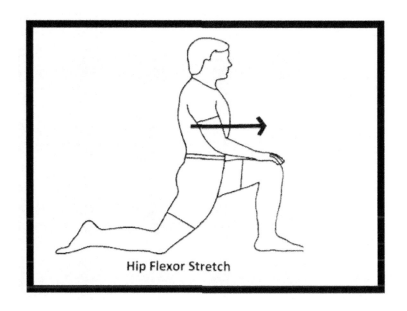

Hip Flexor Stretch

Chapter 12. Rounded shoulders + Uneven shoulders + uneven shoulder height

Have you ever noticed you are standing in front of a mirror and find that one side of your shoulder is rolled forward and possibly the same shoulder is at lower height compared to the other if yes then let's do one more check by checking sideways our shoulder positions.

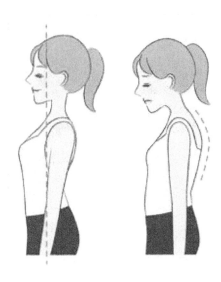

If one of your shoulder has a curve in the back side and the shoulder joint sits forward after looking sideways and the other side is straight and your back looks straight then you have an asymmetrical posture. The side with a curve in the back has strong muscles in the front side which is causing your shoulder to pull forward and weak back muscles and it will be viceversa on the other side. The shoulder which sits forward has strong chest muscles especially the pec minor pulling your shoulder forward and down, the same side will have strong abdominal muscles especially the external oblique muscle and the other side will have strong back muscles that is latissimus dorsi .

Correcting uneven shoulders and rounded shoulders.

There are two cases where both the shoulders are rounded and are pulled forward in that case stretching the chest muscles will be an easy fix but it gets more complicated when it comes to uneven rounded shoulders with uneven height.

Let say you have the right side shoulder rounded or is rolling forward and is on lower side then you need to stretch the right side chest + external oblique muscles and have to strengthen the right side back muscles and on left side you have to stretch the lats and strengthen the pecs + external oblique muscles once you done with stretching and strengthening you must do plank exercise so that your nervous system undergoes the changes that are done.

If you have uneven shoulder height it's most likely that you also have muscle imbalances in your legs that are difficult to identify. It's better to have muscle imbalance checks in your legs also since correcting imbalances in your legs automatically corrects the muscle imbalance in your upper body to some extent.

Chapter 13. Understanding and correcting uneven pecs, uneven traps, uneven lats and shoulders.

Thumb rule if you have muscle imbalances in any part of your body is that if you have imbalances in your chest you will have imbalances in your shoulders, traps and back muscles. If you have understood the posterior and anterior oblique slings then it will become easier for you to identify the weak and strong muscles. Now suppose your right side chest is stronger and the reason is that you are a right hand dominant person and you never stretch your body muscles then the stronger right side chest muscle keeps on getting stronger and stronger. Strong right side chest muscles pull your shoulder blade or scapula forward and make your shoulder height uneven and then your traps also become uneven and at the same time your lats muscle also gets lengthened on the right side back muscles becomes weak.

Correction

Stretch the strong right side chest muscle and at the same time stretch the lats muscles on the left side. Traps are the muscles where you will see the difference immediately since traps muscle is connected to both chest and lats and traps will start getting balanced. Strengthening the weak left side chest muscle and right side lats muscle helps your nervous system to balance out your body, doing this stretching and strengthening exercises will balance your body quickly. Once you start noticing the changes and feel your body balanced then you can stop these exercises.

CHAPTER 14. UNDERSTANDING AND CORRECTING LATERAL PELVIC TILT AND TWISTED CORE.

Have you ever felt or noticed that your body is twisted or you feel that you are losing balance of your body and fall down and you are completely fine mentally, it's just your body is not allowing you to stand properly.

Signs of Lateral pelvic tilt and twisted core.

1) When you sit folding your legs or in a squatting position your upper body rotates.
2) Uneven body mass on one side of your waist and tightness on one side.
3) Uneven rib expansion while breathing.
4) Back pain around the sacroiliac joint.
5) Weak core muscles and difficulty in activating core.

Correction

The most important muscle that needs to be addressed here is the iliopsoas muscle that is connected to spine and imbalance in this muscle leads to spinal misalignment causing rotation in the hips and the upper body (Thoracic body).

So as per the thumb rule for muscle imbalance if one side of your waist is stronger lets say the left side then the right side will be weak causing lateral pelvic tilt.

Lateral pelvic tilt has one side strong quadratus lumborum and iliopsoas muscles and the other side will be weak. Stretching these strong muscles and strengthening the same group of muscles on the weaker side will help to balance out the hips and prevent the upper body from twisting.

CHAPTER 15. TRAINING THE NERVOUS SYSTEM WITH STRETCHING AND STRENGTHENING EXERCISES

How to train your Nervous system ? Your nervous system does not understand your language but it will understand with the help of exercises. Hope you now know the reciprocal inhibition concept, if you are stretching any of the stronger muscles once you identified the muscle imbalance you should always activate or contract the opposite muscles. It's like telling your nervous system to take out the strength from the strong muscles and put it in the weak muscles. So whenever you're stretching the strong muscles you are elongating the muscle and since you're activating the opposite muscles your opposite muscles will become shorter or contracted leading to proper balance of your muscles on both sides.

All the muscle imbalance that occurs it starts from the lower body Any muscle imbalance in the lower body i.e legs and pelvic will be the root cause of muscle imbalance in the upper body if you have right side chest stronger or bigger that means you have strong hip flexors on the left (you can correlate with the myo-fascial slings.)

Below Exercises will help you in fixing asymmetrical posture (Eg. for Right side chest bigger than left side or if you have left side lats muscle stronger then right side or even if you feel you have one leg shorter than the other) (Exercises must be done in sequence as provided below)

Isolated stretch of lower body first and then upper body muscles.

1) Gently Stretch Left side Hip flexors and Adductors.
2) Aggressively Stretch Right side glutes and vastus lateralis muscle.
3) Gently Stretch Left side Quadratus Lumborum , Iliosoas, internal obliques and Lats .
4) Aggressively Stretch right side external oblique muscles , chest muscles and biceps muscle

.

Strengthening Exercise sequence.

1) Strengthen left side glutes and vastus lateralis muscles.
2) Strengthen Right side Adductors.
3) Strengthen right side Lats, internal oblique and Quadratus lumborum.

4) Strengthen left side external oblique, chest and bicep muscles.

5) Finally strengthen the core muscle with Plank exercise (Most important exercise to correct posture permanently)

Exercise Gallery

Myofascial release Hamstrings

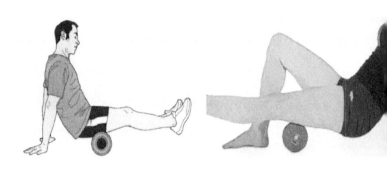

Notes: Use Foam roller in the beginning and lacrosse ball or tennis ball can be used as you progress in your exercises. Use a foam roll for the first ten days.

While myofascial release exercise concentrate on breath in and breathe out and activate the antagonist muscles knee extensors or hip flexors. Make sure to activate the core muscles while performing any exercises.

Hamstring wall stretch

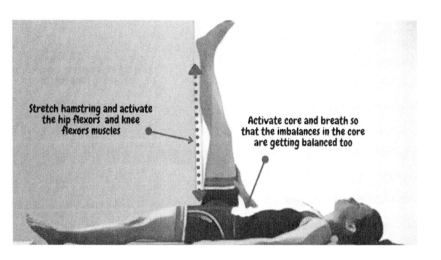

Stretch hamstring and activate the hip flexors and knee flexors muscles

Activate core and breath so that the imbalances in the core are getting balanced too

Myofascial release Glutes

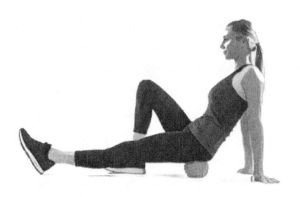

Foam roller, lacrosse ball and tennis ball can be used to release hip flexors.

Stretching Glutes

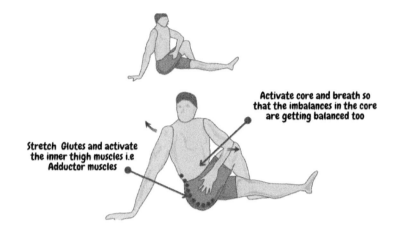

Myofascial release Abductors

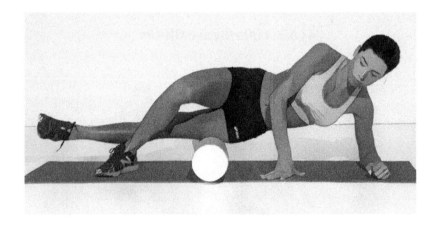

Foam roller, lacrosse ball and tennis ball can be used to release hip flexors.

Abductors Stretch

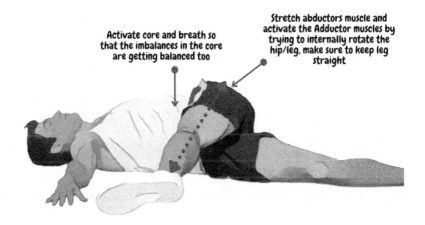

Activate core and breath so that the imbalances in the core are getting balanced too

Stretch abductors muscle and activate the Adductor muscles by trying to internally rotate the hip/leg, make sure to keep leg straight

Myofascial release Hip flexors

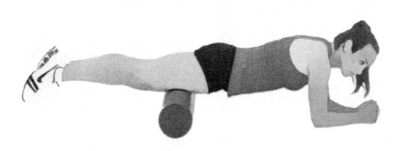

Foam roller, lacrosse ball and tennis ball can be used to release hip flexors

Hip flexors stretch

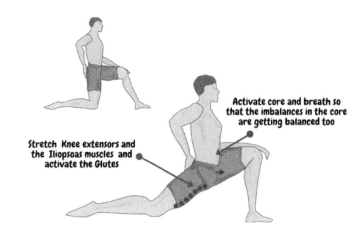

Stretch Knee extensors and the Iliopsoas muscles and activate the Glutes

Activate core and breath so that the imbalances in the core are getting balanced too

Myofascial release adductors

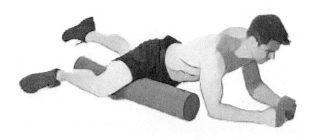

Foam roller can be used to release the adductors

Adductors stretch

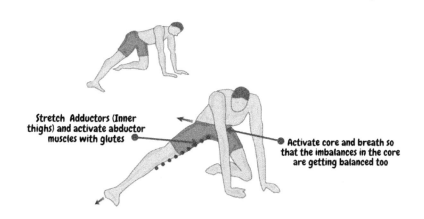

Stretch Adductors (Inner thighs) and activate abductor muscles with glutes

Activate core and breath so that the imbalances in the core are getting balanced too

Myofascial release Pecs/chest

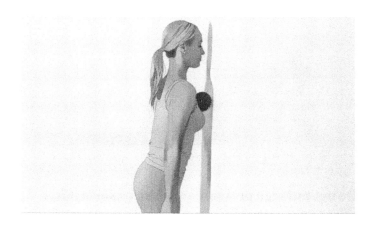

Lacrosse ball or tennis ball can be used to release pecs

Pecs/chest stretch

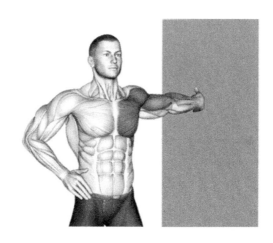

Myofascial release Lats

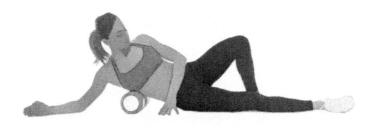

Note: Do not put high pressure on muscles since it is connected to your ribs.
Foam roller, soft tennis and lacrosse ball can be used to release lats.

Lats stretch

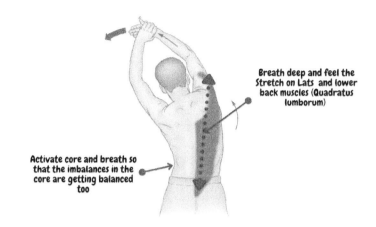

Breath deep and feel the Stretch on Lats and lower back muscles (Quadratus lumborum)

Activate core and breath so that the imbalances in the core are getting balanced too

Myofascial release traps

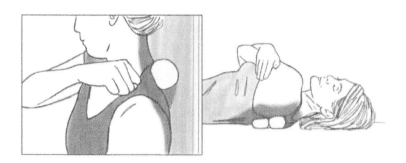

Lacrosse ball or tennis ball can be used to release traps

Traps stretch

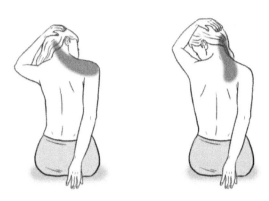

Integrated stretch for External obliques/ adductors

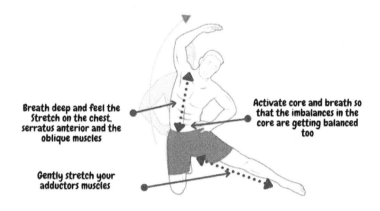

Breath deep and feel the Stretch on the chest, serratus anterior and the oblique muscles

Activate core and breath so that the imbalances in the core are getting balanced too

Gently stretch your adductors muscles

Above stretch is an great example of stretching your entire anterior oblique sling and is recommended only after you do the isolated individual stretching exercises

Chapter 16. Mastering the plank

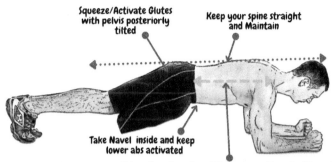

Squeeze/Activate Glutes with pelvis posteriorly tilted

Keep your spine straight and Maintain

Take Navel inside and keep lower abs activated

Take a Deep breath and De-compress the spine(Elongating the spine) and while breathing out try to take your Navel/lower abs towards the spine (Making the core muscle stronger)

Now once you do all the stretching exercises it is very important to do the plank exercise. By doing all the above exercises, it allows the core muscle transverse abdominis to activate to its full potential, since you have minimized the muscle imbalances in other areas now it's time for the transverse abdominis to align the spine, by straightening/decompressing the spine. Most important while doing plank exercise is that your spine should be straight, you should tilt the pelvis posteriorly by activating the glutes and you should take your navel/lower abs towards the spine. Always keep your navel towards your spine. While breathing in take a deep breath so that you feel like you are elongating/decompressing/straightening your spine and while breathing out try to compress your lower abs further and once you exhale keep the position for a few seconds. Start doing the plank exercise daily and start with low intensity/lower time and can increase the intensity as you progress.

CHAPTER 17. CONCLUSION

From this book we understand the working of the human body and by understanding the different Muscle slings we can say that the human body is designed to work in integration and all muscles in our body are connected with each other, if there is one muscle also weak or strong then the entire muscular slings are affected and this causes poor posture and muscle imbalances. But since we now know the science behind it, even if we go through bad posture we can correct the imbalances by doing the self assessment of the body. We can strengthen the weak muscles and Stretch the strong muscles in order to create equal balance of muscles for the process of improving the posture. We can call this the human biomechanics optimization process.

Disclaimer

The information in any of our handouts, e-books, written material, whether provided in hardcopy or digitally (together 'Material') is for general information purposes and nothing contained in it is, or is intended to be construed as advice. It does not take into account your individual health, medical, physical or emotional situation or needs. It is not a substitute for medical attention, treatment, examination, advice, treatment of existing conditions or diagnosis and is not intended to provide a clinical diagnosis nor take the place of proper medical advice from a fully qualified medical practitioner. You should, before you act or use any of this information, consider the appropriateness of this information having regard to your own personal situation and needs. You are responsible for consulting a suitable medical professional before using any of the information or materials contained in our Material or accessed through our website, before trying any treatment or taking any course of action that may directly or indirectly affect your health or well being.

About The Author

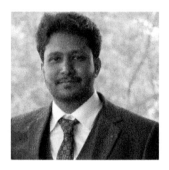

Rangnath Gouda (Posture Guru) is the posture correction expert who helps people facing postural problems He also provides online consultation where he shares and demonstrates the exercises during his consultation. If you are looking for a posture guru you can mail him on postureguru7@gmail.com

Learn more about Rangnath @ https://posture-guru.com

One Last Thing.

If you enjoyed this book or found it useful I'd be very grateful if you'd post a short review on Amazon. Your support really does make a difference and I read all the reviews personally so I can get your feedback and make this book even better.

Printed in Great Britain
by Amazon